Stress
And
Your Health

Recognize the Signs, Symptoms and Adverse Effects Over Time

RON KNESS

Copyright © 2016 Ron Kness

All rights reserved.

ISBN-13: 978-1539766070

ISBN-10: 1539766071

Contents

Disclaimer

We hope you enjoy reading our report however we do suggest you read our disclaimer. All the material written in this report is provided for informational purposes only and is general in nature.

Every person is a unique individual and what has worked for some or even many may not work for you. Any information perceived as advice by must be considered in light of your own particular set of circumstances.

The author or person sharing this information does not assume any responsibility for the accuracy or outcome of your use of the content.

Every attempt has been made to provide well researched and up to date content at the time of writing. Now all the legalities have been taken care of, please enjoy the content.

Introduction

While the word "stress" has many different meanings, as discussed in this publication it refers to the health condition which is all but endemic in modern society. The human body and mind and all its sub-systems developed to deal with the challenges of much more primitive circumstances than we live in now.

Our rapid-response "fight or flight" response system enabled our species to outperform and out-think our way past all others. Collectively our incredible brains have allowed us to live today in a manner that does not require us to engage in the type of activities that made our stress hormones a major asset.

Unfortunately, our physiology has not kept pace with our intellectual development and there is no magic switch to turn off or at least turn down our survival responses. Today, in civilized societies, we encounter a different manner of struggles and challenges.

Even though these situations may not actually be life or death in nature, because of the emotion we attach to our various actions, our minds perceive them as such, and react accordingly.

For many or most people, their bodies and mind are in a constant state of heightened anxiety due to the continually elevated levels of stress hormones in their system. This is chronic stress and its symptoms are broad, varied and can ultimately even be fatal.

We are taught so many things that enable us to live in a social environment with our fellow humans, but too many of us lack knowledge of how to deal with the pressure and stress this can apply. Inability to deal with the causes of stress leads to increased stress and inability to deal with the symptoms of stress can make life seem not worth living.

This publication details some of the signs and symptoms of chronic stress and their damaging effects on our minds and bodies. If you feel stress is negatively impacting your life, make changes. Reduce the causes, or learn to cope with them more appropriately to lessen the impact on you. Seek help if necessary.

Stress and Your Health

Stress has become a very common, misused and misunderstood word in this modern day era. In the physical world, everything has its stress point. This "stress point" refers to the limit of force that a certain material can possibly withstand without being damaged.

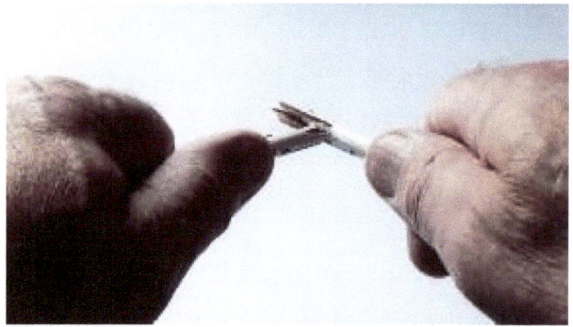

If a material or object is subjected to an amount of force that is beyond its stress point it will most likely be damaged or at least have a reduced ability to survive any more pressure in the future.

The same thing can also be true of the human mind and body. Stress is a fact of life for almost everyone.

Some stress can be very positive, as it keeps people motivated and helps them to grow physically, mentally and emotionally.

Humans can usually deal with stress as long as there are periods of recovery from that stress and healthy ways for dealing with it.

When a person is continually subjected to stress that is beyond their perceived ability to cope, they will begin to exhibit signs and symptoms of chronic stress. Our minds and bodies are not capable of dealing with its cumulative effects all the time.

As humans are not machines, the types, levels and intensity of stress that can be endured by individuals will vary widely. What one person considers stressful may not even be a problem for another.

It has been said that at least 25% of the American population is experiencing "extreme stress".

Individuals operating at that level of stress will certainly be operating at a reduced capacity and struggling to achieve their required productivity levels.

Unless they take steps to mitigate their stressors or ability to deal with them, the problems will worsen along with their ability to perform. Obviously this has a cumulative effect on the productivity of the nation as a whole.

It is sadly ironic that some respondents of the survey nominated the poor economy as a cause of the mounting tension and pressure that they experience on a daily basis which leads them to suffer their extreme levels of stress.

Mild to moderate levels of stress can be beneficial to a person as it sharpens the ability to think while also boosting the physical responses to situations that warrant high levels of performance like athletic competitions and business presentations.

But, if people are chronically stressed over health problems, financial woes or daily irritations like traffic jams, the person's natural fight or flight response will rarely subside.

Signs of Stress to Watch Out For

It is normal for everyone to experience a certain amount of stress in their lives. In fact, since our prehistoric origins, the stress response has been vital for motivating us to react during times of crisis.

Today, we are not literally dealing with "hunt or be hunted" on a regular basis; although, there are certainly days within our current lifestyles that may feel that way!

Our stress hormones can help us to meet strict timelines, and deal with situations we find difficult within our daily lives.

Physical

The physical way we experience stress can vary. Some individuals become extremely irritable with their family members or coworkers.

Others describe a vice-like tension of tightness felt within their chest or shoulders that make it hard to breathe. Numerous people report cardiovascular issues, such as a racing heart, elevated blood pressure and profuse sweating.

Some individuals suffer excruciating headaches or joint and muscle stiffness.

Gastrointestinal issues may be experienced as severe stomach pains and diarrhea. Stress and negative emotions often go hand in hand with poor physical health.

Experiencing emotional stress jump starts the production of cortisol and if this happens on regular basis the excess amount of cortisol will begin to break down the body's neurological, gastrointestinal, musculoskeletal and immune system.

Emotional

Often, it is the emotional side of stress that we initially experience. It is our body's way of warning us that "hey, I'm not ok here...pay attention."

Unfortunately, many people have become accustomed to ignoring the seriousness of messages from their inner selves and prefer to self-medicate or deny their stress altogether. This is a dangerous habit to get into.

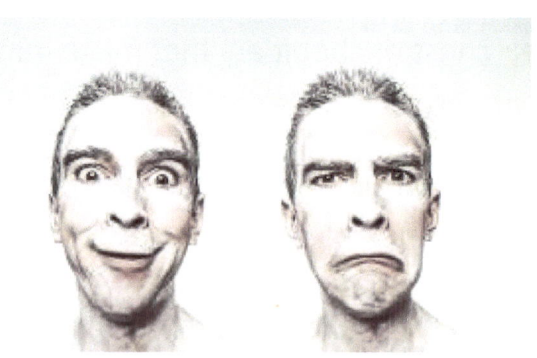

Society has taught us, particularly men, that feeling and especially expressing your feelings is wrong. Denying your feelings will potentially only make things much worse.

Chronic or unrelenting stress, if ignored, can manifest as a physical response in the body in the form of illness or emotionally as depression.

If left unchecked, stress can be very damaging to a person's health. This will compound the problem, which will very likely lead to an adverse effect on other aspects of a person's life.

If you find yourself experiencing some or any of these signs, pause and reflect. Review your life and your priorities to reduce if not eliminate some of your stressors.

Symptoms of stress such as acne, bald patches and dry skin may be visible and obvious. Although the mental and emotional damage may itself not be visible, their effects on self and loved ones usually are.

If your stress levels are left untreated, you are likely to ultimately suffer from even more serious health problems such as heart disease, obesity and depression.

Learning How to Cope

Many people think that being stressed is completely normal and many brag about how stressed they are. After all, everybody's experiencing it! Unfortunately, stress has very insidious ways of wreaking havoc on an individual.

It can have adverse effects not just on the person's physical looks, but it can also affect their emotional and mental aspects.

Health professionals, community groups and governments encourage everybody to embrace healthy coping mechanisms that give them a better fighting chance against stress.

A body in good physical health is far better able to deal with the consequences of excess stress.

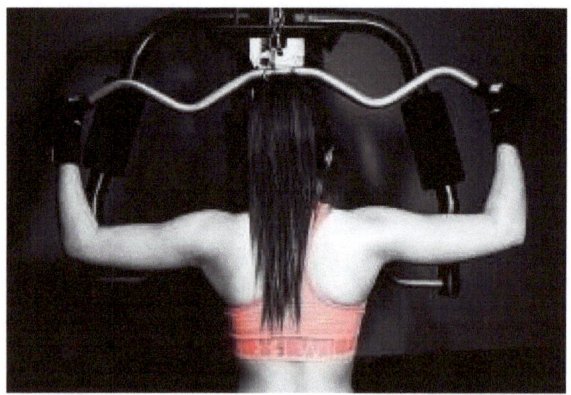

If you are excessively overweight or underweight, your body will be more adversely affected and slower to recover. Make yourself aware of the symptoms and dangers of stress, how it can affect you and how you can mitigate the impacts on your life.

Notice your behavior. Pay attention to things, situations and people who you constantly find triggering your stress response.

Once you are aware of your stressors, you will be able to recognize them in advance and take the appropriate steps. Possibly, you can avoid certain stressors altogether.

Other times, you can desensitize yourself by planning in advance.

If you have pre-existing medical issues such as chronic pain or cardiovascular problems, you may notice that they flare up more or increase dramatically when you are stressed out in particular situations.

Try incorporating some exercise into your day. Punch or scream into a pillow if necessary. The important thing is to acknowledge and release these pent up emotions.

Stuffing them down deep or compartmentalizing them may make you feel better temporarily; however, it will do you absolutely no good in the future and could potentially make you very sick in the meantime.

Monitor and Act

While no symptom in isolation can be taken as a diagnosis, clusters of symptoms should be taken as a warning.

Review your day-to-day actions, monitor your feelings and reactions, and if chronic or ongoing stress is affecting your life, make changes or seek help before it gets worse.

Symptoms of Chronic Stress

As stress-related illness seems almost endemic today, there is no shortage of data for health researchers to study.

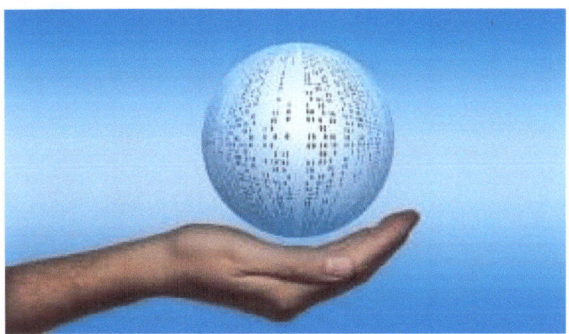

This has enabled health professionals to diagnose excessive stress as an illness, based on the symptoms displayed by a patient. It has also allowed them to predict the areas of human health that are most likely to be compromised as a result of stress.

While the range and intensity of symptoms can vary from patient to patient, some symptoms are closely correlated to chronic stress. When these occur as a cluster a diagnosis of chronic stress is even more likely.

Heart

Research shows that employees who are frequently exposed to high levels of work-related stress are at a higher risk of being diagnosed with cardiovascular disease. This risk is also often compounded by an individual's bad lifestyle habits such as eating processed foods, smoking cigarettes and drinking alcoholic beverages.

Unfortunately, these poor lifestyle choices are often made and increased as coping mechanisms to deal with stress. Long-term, these habits add to the cumulative stresses on the individuals physical and emotional state.

Stress causes massive depletion of the mineral magnesium, which is essential for muscle relaxation.

Tests have shown that a very large percentage of the adult population are magnesium-deficient, which very likely has a strong correlation to those affected by chronic stress.

As the heart is a muscle it is dependent on adequate magnesium for proper and healthy function. Current research is exploring the possible link between low magnesium levels and heart attacks.

Acute stress, such as may occur to people who are experiencing the sudden death of a loved one, a natural disaster or extreme accident may also lead to stress-induced cardiomyopathy. These cases may seem rare but are well-documented.

Thankfully, increased awareness means that professional emotional support is offered far more now than before, with better outcomes for those affected.

Pancreas

People who are chronically stressed have a high tendency to indulge in sugary, feel-good foods. A stressed mindset is not conducive to mindful dietary habits.

Under continued stress a person is far more likely to be looking for highly processed convenience food; for both comfort and speed. Also, the actual stress itself can cause elevated levels of blood glucose.

Unfortunately, if this stress-induced increase in blood glucose is compounded by poor eating habits an individual may sooner or later increase their weight gain.

The combination of obesity and difficulty managing blood glucose levels are leading indicators of being diagnosed with Type 2 diabetes.

Stomach Problems

Do you feel like your stomach has been invaded by butterflies? This is a normal reaction to many stressful or fearful circumstances.

However, if this feeling persists long after the stressful situation is over then you should start monitoring your feelings throughout the day. Persistent feelings of being stressed or pressured at times when the actual stress trigger has long passed is cause for concern.

A regular stomach ache is one of the many symptoms that can be experienced by an individual who is suffering from stress.

The nervous system, which includes the brain, is connected to our gut and this is why mental stress adversely affects the GI tract.

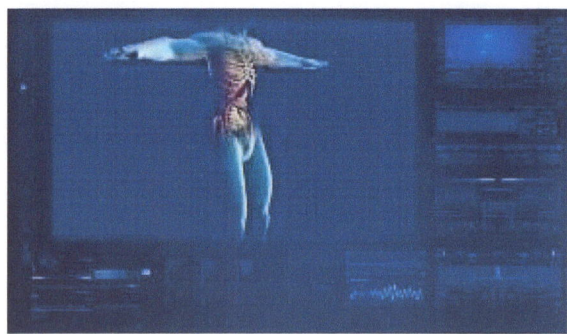

Chronic stress can ultimately lead to symptoms of irritable bowel syndrome. Continually feeling pressured can cause poor bowel elimination routines. If the cause is left unchecked, this could escalate into other gastric problems.

Many cases of gastrointestinal disorders such as diarrhea, constipation and irritable bowel syndrome have been linked to stress. This shows how our brain and our gut are so interconnected to each other.

Exercise is the best and safest remedy for stress-induced vomiting, nausea, diarrhea and constipation.

It may seem like the last thing that you want to do when you have a stomach ache but exercise helps boost the production of endorphins that are responsible for that "feel-good" experience. This means exercise will provide relief via both physical and emotional channels.

Depending on the kind of stomach problem you have, your doctor will most likely prescribe you some stool softeners, anti-nausea meds or some over-the-counter drugs. You will also be advised to make dietary changes such as increased fiber intake.

Fiber can help restore those stress-ravaged bacteria in your gut to make you feel better. While these short-term solutions may be necessary to 'soldier on', the symptoms should also be taken as a wakeup call to take action to reduce, prevent and better deal with stress.

Gastroenterologists will often advise their patients to find ways to better deal with their stress early in their treatment protocols. They recommend that their patients indulge in relaxing activities in order to lessen the stress and reverse the syptoms of it.

This is because doctors know that bowel-specific medications will not be fully effective unless something is also done to reduce the patient's stress levels.

Skin

Psoriasis, eczema, and other skin inflammations are often linked to prolonged exposure to stress.

Our skin is the largest immune organ and stress is a common cause of lowered immune system levels. Therefore, if a person is stressed their immune system also suffers which manifests through skin inflammations.

In most cases of skin diseases that have been brought on by stress, reducing stress levels have also been found to rapidly improve a person's skin condition.

Acne

Acne can also be a symptom of another disease such as rosacea, Cushing's Syndrome or polycystic ovarian syndrome (PCOS). However, chronic exposure to stress can also lead to the overproduction of the sex hormone androgen, resulting in acne and other skin problems.

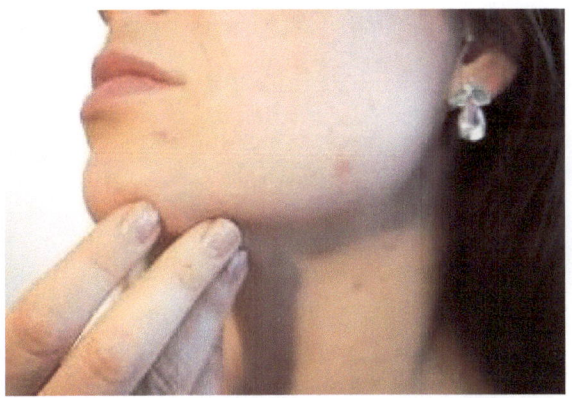

Stress causes excessive hormone production combined with a reduced healing ability, meaning you may experience the same types of skin problems you did as a teenager.

Hair

While hair loss can be a sign of another more serious condition such as alopecia areata and telogen effluvium, it can also be one of the most common symptoms of stress.

Hair loss will be most likely to happen three to six months after a traumatic experience such as losing a loved one or losing a job.

When a person is exposed to highly-stressful events their androgen hormone production will be imbalanced, possibly resulting in temporary hair loss. Sticking to a balanced diet is important at times of high stress to give the body every possible assistance for healing and repair.

You may often hear people say that stress is turning their hair to grey. Stress can speed up this process especially if you are already genetically predisposed to having grey hair.

During periods of prolonged stress, an individual's white blood cells may attack their hair follicles thereby putting a halt to hair growth which is also called a "resting phase".

This is when too much hair is lost when being washed or combed. There are also cases when stress can severely affect an individual in a condition called trichotillomania, which causes them to have an irresistible urge to pull out their hair.

Menstrual Cycle Problems

Missed and delayed periods can be a sign of stress in women. In severe cases, some women may suffer from secondary amenorrhea which leads to a complete stop of the menstrual cycle.

Other women still experience regular menstrual periods but many complain of dysmenorrhea that is twice as painful when they're feeling excessive stress.

Bruxism

Have you heard about people chewing over their day's stressors during their sleep? Some stressed individuals grind their teeth while they are sleeping. There are also those who clench their jaws without even noticing it during the daytime.

Teeth grinding and jaw clenching can damage a person's teeth or cause tooth and jaw pains. If you are experiencing these symptoms, seriously consider consulting your health care provider and your dentist. In addition to working to reduce the root cause, you may need to use a mouth guard or other precautionary measure.

Eye Twitching

Although there have been no studies yet to definitely prove it many people complain about eye twitching when they're fatigued or stressed.

Decreased Libido

It is common for people who are under a great deal of stress or feeling exhausted to have no desire in the bedroom. This can be frustrating for your spouse or partner as well. If you are suffering from a general lack of libido possibly caused by stress, it is essential to confide in your partner so that they can lend a sympathetic ear and not take it personally.

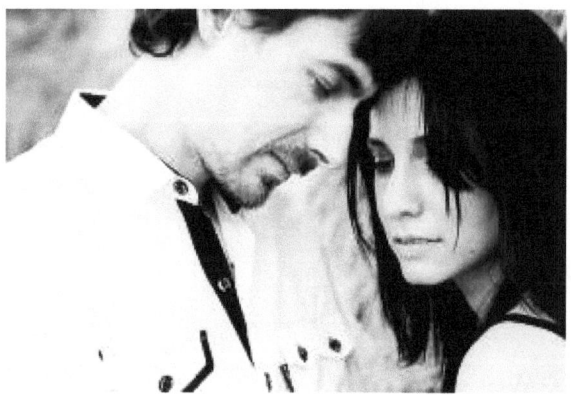

Muscle Tightness

Tensed muscles are common indications of stress. This can further lead to muscle spasms which can cause great pain.

Stress causes magnesium depletion in the body and without magnesium the muscles cannot relax, putting them in a state of near-constant contraction. If muscle tightness is not reduced or eliminated through massage, check that your vitamin and mineral intake is adequate.

Weird Dreams

Many people complain about having weird dreams at night whenever they are subjected to too much pressure during the day. Juggling between too many responsibilities and unfinished tasks during daytime may mean your mind is working even while you sleep.

Obviously if this is the case you are not getting the quality rest your mind and body craves and needs.

Insomnia and Difficulty Sleeping

Is worrying about the past, present or future causing you sleepless nights? Maybe it's the complete opposite for you and it takes everything just to drag yourself out of bed each morning? Perhaps you spend your day counting down the hours until you can reunite with your fluffy duvet? Sleeping difficulties can lead to feeling extremely lethargic.

It is hard to be ultra-productive when you suffering from fatigue and walking around in a daze.

Chronic stress can cause a horrible marriage of both; feeling drugged and unmotivated when clarity is needed, and churning wakefulness when you should be sleeping.

People who are subjected to too much stress can often find themselves having difficulty switching off their thinking and this can make sleep very elusive for them. Ruminating stressful thoughts, studying and watching TV can keep the brain active thereby making it harder for an individual to fall asleep.

Wind down by meditating or listening to soothing music to relax your brain and allow sleep to embrace you naturally. Developing healthy sleeping habits such as avoiding caffeine and other stimulants a few hours before bedtime is also a much better option than relying solely on sleeping pills that can do more harm than good.

Effects of Chronic Stress

For several years, with the help of advanced lab techniques, experts have tried their best to unlock the complex picture of how chronic stress causes such a profound and damaging impact on the human body. Here are some of the findings from different studies relative to chronic stress and its impact on human health.

Telomerase

At the end of each chromosome are caps which are called telomeres. These look like shoelace tips and were found by experts to shorten every time the cell divides. When these telomeres become too small the cell will eventually die. Our bodies also produce an enzyme called telomerase that helps lengthen the telomeres.

Telomerase levels were found to increase with the help of several stress reduction techniques, including meditation and Yoga. On the contrary, chronic exposure to stress can lead to premature telomere contraction.

In other words, exposure to high levels of stress can speed up cell aging which also further increases the likelihood of being diagnosed with diabetes, arthritis and many other neurodegenerative diseases such as dementia.

Cortisol

Being chronically exposed to increased levels of cortisol has been found to trigger insulin resistance and such an occurrence is also a known precursor to diabetes. Doctors who regularly work with cancer sufferers also found out that cortisol inhibits the production of a tumor suppression gene. This finding has lead experts to believe that having high levels of cortisol in the body can speed up the progression of cancer cells.

A group of Dutch researchers conducted a study which followed 800 participants aged 65 years and older. At the start of the study, researchers identified who among the participants had the highest levels of cortisol. After six years, they found out that these groups of people were at higher risk of dying from a cardiovascular disease compared to study participants who only had low levels of cortisol. The same risk factor is also expected to apply even to those study participants who showed no signs of heart problems at the start of the study.

Neuropeptide Y

Chronic stress has also been linked to the accumulation of deep belly fat. This is because when an individual is under stress, the neurotransmitter NPY or neuropeptide Y will send signals to the abdomen telling it to store fat and to find more cells that will be converted into fat.

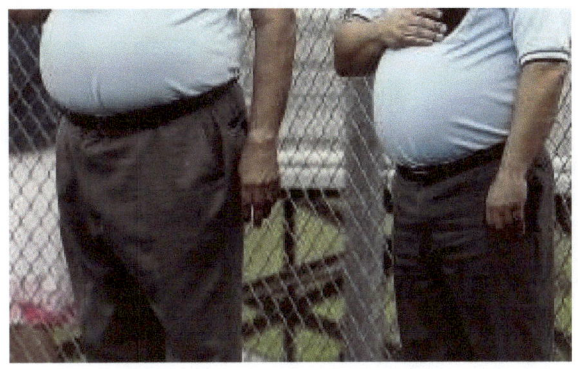

This finding coincides with the evolutionary fact that the body finds it easier to convert those fats found in the belly into the energy that is needed in order to fight or outrun a predator. Fat is stored in the midriff as this area does not contain the muscles which are needed for fight and flight, such as arms, legs and buttocks.

A combination of a stress-driven society and a lifestyle that has much less high-intensity energy expenditure goes a long way towards explaining why there is such a prevalence of belly fat in modern western societies. It also explains why belly fat is so easy to put on and so hard to take off.

Stress and Its Adverse Effects on the Brain

Do you often find yourself frantically looking for car keys or phone every morning? This scenario is no longer unusual for many of us.

In fact, we often blame our memory when we find that we have left important documents at home or when we misplace some of our files in the office.

These things may occur because our brains sometimes just do not have the capacity to cope with all the stressful events we are facing each day.

Unfortunately, when we forget something there is always that added pressure to be able to find what we lost or misplaced. In turn, our brain is exposed to even more stress and must double its efforts. Even though it's already overloaded state caused the memory lapse it now has to perform under even greater immediate load.

Sometimes it is impossible to remember the required detail at this stressed level.

How many times have you remembered something shortly after the pressure is removed? As stress levels reduce, the brain moves into more proper functioning and seemingly effortlessly pops up information.

This small example shows clearly how strongly our brain function is adversely affected by stress. Just as importantly, it should remind us of the need to reduce stress to have our minds function at their best for us.

Stress can adversely affect an individual's brain, specifically the part that regulates metabolism and emotions. Researchers have found that it is not only major or life-changing individual traumatic events can have negative impacts to the brain.

All the stressful events that people have been exposed to in their lifetime can also have a cumulative effect.

While this is in itself disturbing knowledge, it is reassuring to know that reduction in stress and its positive effects are also cumulative. Any successful efforts at lowering stress will have beneficial flow on effects.

Stress and the Prefrontal Cortex of the Brain

One study had 100 healthy people as participants who provided plenty of information about the stressful and traumatic events they experienced in their lives.

All the participants of the study shared their experiences about divorce, grief, loss of job and loss of property. The brain imaging system revealed that the prefrontal cortex part of the brain is the most vulnerable to the impacts of stress.

Importantly, the prefrontal cortex is the part of the brain responsible for maintaining insulin, glucose levels, emotions, self-control and other physiological functions.

Stress Affects Specific Parts of the Brain

During brain imaging researchers were able to discover that different stressful events also affect different regions of the brain. For example, the part of the brain responsible for emotions is greatly affected by recent traumatic events such as job loss and medical diagnosis.

When this specific region of the brain shrinks significantly an individual will tend to increasingly lose touch with his emotions and even act inappropriately. In very real ways this can also affect how an individual interacts with other people.

On the other hand, when an individual suffers from a serious illness such as cancer or when a person has lost a loved one the mood centers of the brain are acutely affected. In turn, the person's reward and pleasure centers become distorted.

When these stressful events adversely impact the brain volume the person will become progressively more vulnerable to the symptoms of depression and anxiety.

Chronic Stress Affects our Coping Skills

Another finding of the study indicated that being exposed to chronic stress may deteriorate some areas of the brain in a very gradual manner. This gradual deterioration is almost imperceptible so it can be that only when the person experiences a highly-stressful or traumatic event that the cumulative effect of stress become magnified.

This can then manifest in a person's poor coping skills during times of adversity. Had there not been the deterioration due to chronic stress the person would have better been able to cope with the acute emotional trauma.

Knowing how stress impacts the brain should give us the impetus to take steps to mitigate our stress, such as exercising, meditating and practicing other relaxation techniques.

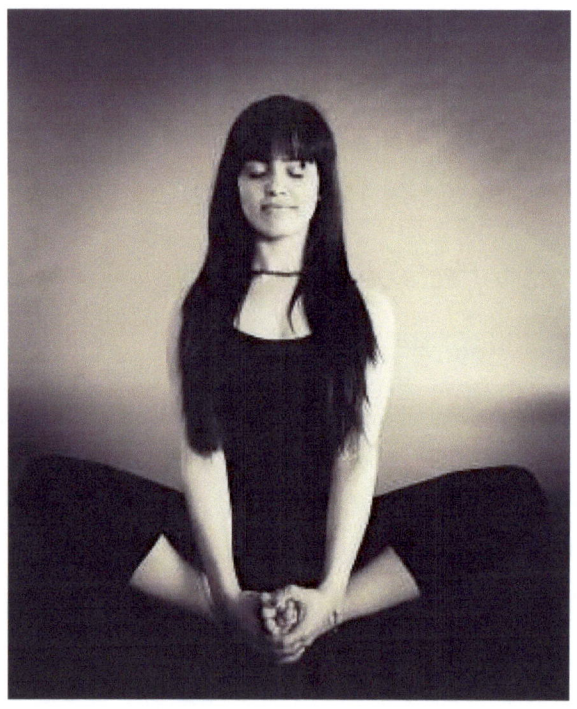

Having that improved capability to cope with stress and reduce its effects will lessen the impact that stress has on our brains.

Another way to diffuse the harmful effects of stress is to maintain positive emotional and social relationships with our loved ones and friends.

These people will serve as our support group in the times when stress becomes too much for us to cope on our own.

Conclusion

At the very least, the information you have gleaned above will have made you realize, just in case you hadn't already, how dangerous chronic stress is to human health and well-being.

Hopefully if you are suffering the effects of stress and felt alone or isolated, you will realize you are one of an untold number of diagnosed and undiagnosed sufferers of chronic stress.

Even more hopefully still, you will have realized that although we all have to live our daily lives, that chronic stress is not inevitable. You can take steps to minimize its terrible impact on yourself. An improved quality of life is optionally available, but of course effort is required.

Be kind to yourself and make yourself the best project for overcoming stress that you can!

In the next chapter, I have included a few of my books that may interest you if you want to further read about stress and how to reduce and control its effects.

Other Relevant Health Books by This Author

If you would like to read more about stress, here is a partial list of titles, CreateSpace links and descriptions:

https://www.createspace.com/6357470

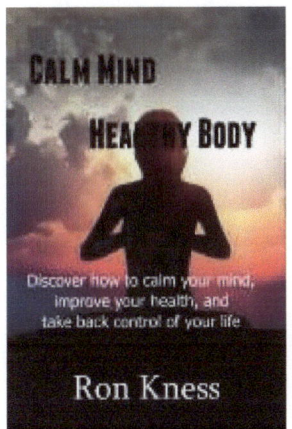

Calm Mind – Healthy Body

Do you ever get the feeling like you're constantly putting out fires? Like life is one massive struggle to stay afloat?

Do you come home from work feeling tired and stressed and without the energy to do anything other than collapse in front of the TV?

Do you always feel like you're just not quite as happy as you think you could/should be?

That's life my friend in today's world. Or at least it's life as many of us have come to know it. In fact though, there's no reason this should necessarily be the case.

The problem is we're always chasing after the gold at the end of the rainbow and in doing so, we end up chasing out tail and take the time to stop and smell the roses.
We're never happy because we're always striving for "the next big thing" and what is coming next.

We're always stressed about what's coming up and we never appreciate what we have here and now until we lose it.

We think the only way to change this is to change our lives. To work harder and longer, which in the end only adds to the problem.

But it's not. The way we change this is from the inside out. We need to change the way we think about our situation and we need to change the way we approach life's problems and the way we enjoy the moment.

And that means taking control of our individual minds.

Once you can do that, you can take back control and you can feel confident, relaxed and happy in the exact same circumstances. Once you can do that, you can start creating the space to actually plot a course and to start changing life for the better. You can stop treading water and actually start swimming.

All very abstract, yes. So far it sounds like a platitude from a bumper sticker.

But stick with me, because this is where the science comes in. And it might just change the way you think about your life, your brain and the interplay between the two.

In this book, we discuss various techniques in which you can use to calm your mind and improve your health.

https://www.createspace.com/6296681

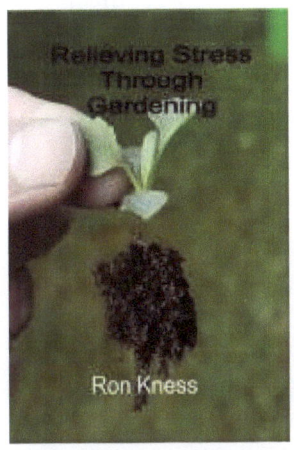

Relieving Stress Through Gardening

Warning: Stress Is Spiraling Dangerously Out of Control and So Is Prescription Drug Abuse

Learn How to Handle Your Stress Through a Natural Solution That Provides Both Mental and Physical Health Benefits!

In "Relieving Stress Through Gardening", you're going to discover an all natural solution that zaps stress and eliminates the need for you to pop pills on a regular basis.

Gardening sounds like a simple activity, but the benefits are both mental and physical in nature. There are vitamins absorbed through the skin from the sun and beneficial bacteria that thrive in the dirt – both of which help diminish your cortisol levels and help you handle whatever comes your way.

In Gardening for Stress Relief, you'll begin to understand...

==> The Scientific Explanation for How Gardening Impacts Your Sleep Cycles and Helps Eliminate Stress Permanently!

==> Why Gardening Trumps Exercise in Helping You Stick to a Program of All Natural Stress Relieving Physical Activity That Sends Cortisol Packing Through Feel Good Hormones!

==> How Gardening Contributes to a Peaceful State of Mind That Carries Over to Your Bedtime Ritual and Removes Stress from Your Sleep Equation!

==> The Precise Way Gardening Puts Your Sleep Cycles Back on Track after They've Been Derailed by Excessive Amounts of Stress!

==> How Gardening Helps Kids Leave the Pressures of the World Behind and Get a Good Night's Sleep!

==> Specific Plants You Can Grow in Your Garden to Help You Relax and Unwind at the End of a Hard Day So You Can Drift Off with Ease!

==> Why Gardening Has Been Called the #1 Sleep Aid that Trumps Prescription Drugs and Contributes to Your Health from Head to Toe!

Once you start gardening, whether it's on a small micro scale or a large plot of land, you'll begin to see immediate changes in the way that you rest each night. You'll be amazed at how the combination of vitamin D, fresh air, peace of mind and low impact physical activity makes you nod off without hesitation.

https://www.createspace.com/6236630

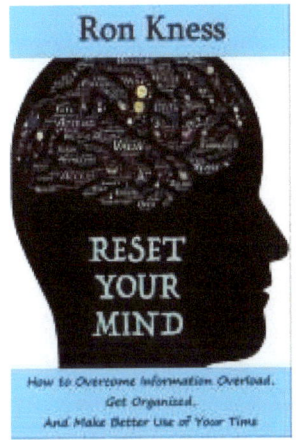

Reset Your Mind

Have you ever thought that maybe you had too much on your plate?

That you'd work better if you had less on your mind?

Imagine how free you'd feel. Much less stressed and able to think clearly for the first time!

Believe it or not, feeling the way you are now is not normal you don't have to be overloaded.

Can You Imagine Working Twice As Fast?

You can by applying what is in our detailed and informative guide that will give you guidance on how YOU can rid yourself of information overload and work more efficiently and effectively.

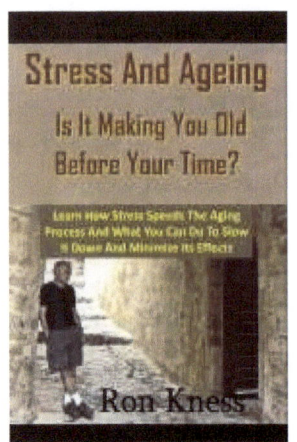

Stress and Ageing

The stress response occurs when external or internal factors cause the body's adrenal glands to put out excess epinephrine, norepinephrine, and cortisol.

These response hormones can result in an increased heart rate, respiratory rate, blood pressure, and blood glucose levels.

A stressor can be anything from having a bad day at the office, relationship issues, physical or emotional distress, financial problems, and a whole host of other things that infiltrate our daily lives, resulting in a stress response.

While stress is normal, too much of it, or too often, can lead to negative effects on your health. In this book we discuss how to recognize stress and how to minimize its effects to keep you from getting old before your time.

About the Author

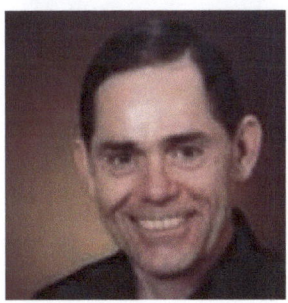

I grew up in Central Minnesota, where my parents owned and operated a fishing resort. Once out of high school I tried a couple of semesters of college, only to quit halfway through the Spring term; I decided at that time that college wasn't for me.

Then I decided to follow my father's previous occupation as an auto mechanic. I graduated from a two-year of vocational training course and worked as a mechanic for five years. While in vocational training, I decided to join the National Guard where I eventually ended up working full-time for 32 years.

So how does all of this relate to writing? In one of my leadership schools, the instructor, who was an English teacher at a juvenile detention center, presented writing to me in a whole new way - a way that started to develop my interest in working with words.

I eventually went back to college on the GI Bill while I

was working and earned my Bachelor's degree in Business Administration. Taking a class or two per semester at night and on weekends took me seven years to complete my degree.

Fast forward about 40 years and I now have published over 75 books on Amazon for Kindle, CreateSpace and other publishing platforms.

Besides my own writing, I also ghostwrite ebooks, reports, articles, blogs and do Kindle conversions for clients on a variety of topics.

Today my wife and I are retired from our careers and live in Gold Canyon, AZ. I now write as a retirement business where you'll find me happily sitting in my office typing away on my laptop as I work on my next book or ghostwriting project . . . that is if we are not traveling on a cruise ship - our new-found mode of travel.